PRAISE FOR
CREATING SACRED SPACE

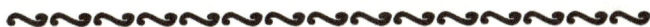

~~~~~~~~~~~~~~~~~~~~~~~~~~~~~

"If you want to read a book with proven strategies to help you get past those obstacles that are holding you back in life, then, this is a MUST READ! Ingrid walks her talk in this inspiring, engaging book that is full of practical tools. If you want to lose the excuses and break negative patterns to get on the path to consistently succeed, then I urge you to get this book! This is highly recommended."

—**LEESA LANDRY**, Author of
The Gift of Divorce

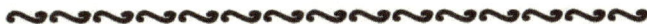

~~~~~~~~~~~~~~~~~~~~~~~~~~~~~

~~~~~~

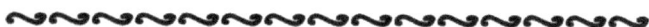

"Creating Sacred Space is an amazing, comprehensive guide to helping anyone greatly improve their lives no matter where you are in your journey. Ingrid is full of wisdom and passion and will make a powerful impact."

—**TRAVON TAYLOR**, international speaker and trainer; author of the bestselling book, *Success Chasing You*

~~~~~~

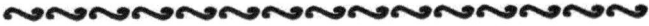

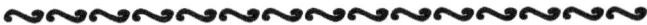

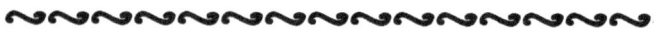

"Creating Sacred Space: A Journey to Self-Healing and Living the Life of Your Dreams! This book provides step by step support for those stuck without a program for spiritual purpose and renewal. I have given copies to clients to help start the process of self-awareness on their journey of healing energy."

—**CALAH BROOKS**, CRA-RT,
Let it go with Reiki

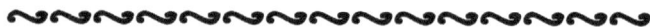

~~~~~~~~~~~~~~~~~~~~~~~~~

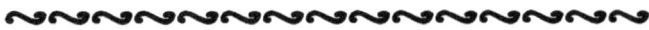

"If you have a desire to experience more clarity in your life and wish to move from pain to passion and purpose, this book is for you. As you follow the recommended exercises, you will connect more deeply with your True Self and will receive the guidance you need to break free from whatever is stopping you from living your best life."

—**MARISA FERRERA**, Women's Empowerment Coach and Author of Best Selling Book: *Magnify Your Magnificence: Your Pathway to the Life & Relationships You Truly Desire*

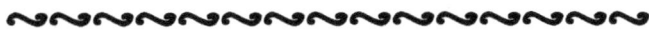

~~~~~~~~~~~~~~~~~~~~~~~~~

CREATING SACRED SPACE

A Journey to Self-Healing
and Living the Life
of Your Dreams!

Ingrid Herbert

GLOBAL WELLNESS MEDIA
Los Angeles—Toronto

COPYRIGHT

CREATING SACRED SPACE:
A Journey to Self-Healing and Living
the Life of Your Dreams!

Copyright © 2019 Ingrid Herbert.

Copyright Use and Public Information

Please contact the author for questions about copyrights or the use of public information.

WellnessToGo.ca/contact

Limits of Liability and Disclaimer of Warranty

The author and publisher shall not be liable for your misuse of this material. This book is strictly for informational and educational purposes.

The views expressed are those of the author.

PUBLISHER

GLOBAL WELLNESS MEDIA
Strategic Edge Innovations Publishing

Los Angeles
340 S Lemon Ave #2027
Walnut, California 91789-2706

Toronto
551 Lakeshore Rd East, S.111
Mississauga, Ontario, L5G 1H0

866.467-9090

GlobalWellnessMedia.com

CREDITS

Book Editor: Emma Steel
Book Design: SEI Publishing
Cover Design: Black Card Books
Illustrations: Envato (Weapedesign)
Manuscript Support: Claire Oxford

ISBN: 978-1-7753487-0-2 (Paperback)
ISBN: 978-0-9863112-7-7 (Digital)

TABLE OF CONTENTS

BOOK 1

BOOK 2

ACKNOWLEDGEMENTS

My heart is filled with gratitude to my mentor and friend Charlene Roycht, my friend and colleague Marisa Meléndez, my friend Angela De Sario, my friend and colleague Rekha Morbia, and my mentor and friend Veronica McCarthy for their support. To my grand-mother for her teachings, insights, and encouragement who put me on this journey from a very young age. To my editor Emma Steel and Claire Oxford for helping to shape the manuscript.

More Than You Know

There are feelings and thoughts that can never truly be expressed through the written and or spoken word

They are not concrete enough to be Comprehended – fully.

In order to give understanding to the one they are being told to and or felt for.

Because of this difficulty, they remain forever in the abstract.

They are emotions which have become symbiotic with the soul.

Unfortunately, you cannot project your feelings

inside another 'Being' and make them feel and see things the way you feel and see them.

The question remains…

How do you convey these feelings to another person?

When all you have are words?

Their frailty is seen when even the slightest gesture or tone may be misunderstood.

Ingrid Herbert

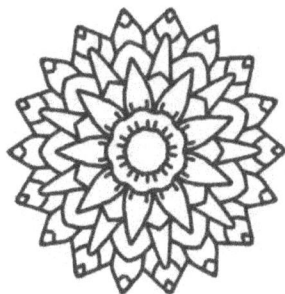

FOREWORD

For many years — I've experienced the very multi-gifted and talented Ingrid's healings. She's an extra-ordinary healer.

In this book she touches upon all the tools to create one's sacred space and nothing more important than getting in touch with your True Self! When your body, mind and soul are aligned — you are unstoppable. And she's so right suggesting one to slow down ... go inwards. That is the key.

Read her book! She has very valuable insights, knowledge and experience to share.

She's been a part of my medical/healing circle for years ... a very good soul !!!

Charlene Roycht
Co-Active Life Coach

ABOUT THE AUTHOR

INGRID HERBERT wears many hats as an expert holistic health practitioner, a mom, a divorcee, and a sole surviving parent. She has challenged herself to experience deeper fulfillment in her passions and to create better life experiences for her clients, her son, and herself.

Her own personal journey to self-healing started in her early 20's after suffering for several years with debilitating health issues. Herbert's health crisis started from the young age of 14 with excruciating menstrual cycles, autoimmune system deficiency, and spinal problems. Doctors experimented on her with different treatments and medications that were temporary fixes but with no lasting solutions.

For close to a decade, she lived in a permanent health crisis, which cost her jobs, friendships, and relationships. She had what she called a half-life.

Eventually, she found her breakthroughs with alternative treatments such as meditation, reiki, and bio-dynamic therapy to name a few, which led her to develop her own personal practice of Sacred Space.

This is one of a few reasons why she writes this

book. These life lessons helped her to learn the secrets to managing overwhelming emotional and physical crisis while continuing to have a healthy positive outlook on life.

Her journey has created the opportunity for her to master the disciplines of living a better quality of life which she has also taught her clients to take back control of their emotions, create breakthroughs in their personal life, health, or career crisis. She gives them the tools to cope in any situation.

Thankfully, she has placed laughter high on the list in her home which she's taken into her career, her motto is "If it's not fun I'm not doing it."

She has taught her son and her clients that fun doesn't always mean you're laughing all the way through it, but it could also mean there is no place you'd rather be than where you are in that moment.

Drawing on 15 years of experience as a holistic health practitioner, she is known for credible and manageable solutions to help individuals with their everyday wellness and lifestyle needs.

Herbert has helped clients find joy in their relationships, more fulfillment in their careers, and transition through terminal illnesses with partners, family, and their own life-changing diagnosis and surgeries.

Many of us go through difficult hardships and challenges within society. Her goal is no matter the circumstances that you are faced with, she wants to help you get the opportunity to live your life fully.

She hopes this book inspires individuals, couples, and families to strive for better health and to live their best lives mentally, physically, spiritually, and emotionally on the planet.

"I've learned that the most important step in anyone's healing is the belief and acceptance of a possible solution."

—INGRID HERBERT

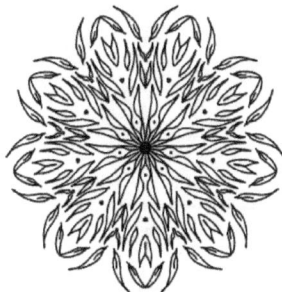

ABOUT THE BOOK

This book offers you solutions to be the best possible version of yourself.

- To live in the NOW with more self-awareness
- To live with more clarity in your daily life experiences
- To get unstuck and overcome emotional setbacks to achieve your goals
- To live a life with deeper satisfaction and more enjoyment from the outcome of your decisions

It will give you the tools, habits, and strategies to heal the body and mind, manage stress, and create personal growth and development.

Are you ready to stop feeling overwhelmed by the multiple decisions that need to be made in all areas of your life? Are you ready to commit to daily disciplines that will transform your failures and setbacks to success? Would you like to learn how to express your negative emotions and thoughts in a more positive way? Are you frustrated that the enjoyment and satisfaction you should be feeling after you've accomplished your goals aren't there? Are you ready to have more passionate connections in your life no matter what your current circumstances are?

LEARN HOW TO...

Finally break the cycle of struggling with the daily issues of overwhelming emotional setbacks, loss of direction, feeling stuck, and just surviving the eat- fight-sleep routine while feeling the lack of something important in your life.

You will experience the power of these tools and techniques to move from an ordinary lifestyle to one that is extraordinary where you feel fulfilled and passionate and where you have a deeper satisfaction and more enjoyment in your day-to-day activities.

This is a powerful system with proven strategies that help you to connect with the best version of yourself. It offers daily disciplines that will transform your failures and setbacks to success. Learn how to express your negative emotions and thoughts in a more positive way. You can finally stop feeling overwhelmed by the multiple decisions that need to be made in all areas of your life. You will uncover the secrets to navigate the day-to-day struggles and get more satisfaction from achieving your goals; you will accelerate your results and transform your life. Eventually, you will master the skills to create the ideal life you've always envisioned for yourself.

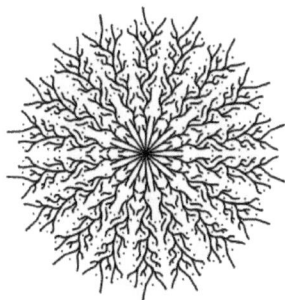

SPECIAL BONUS

**As a special thanks for purchasing
this book, I am offering you
the following bonuses:**

Free download of my tools to
complement your healing journey:

Detox & De-Clutter 101
and
**The Sacred Space Process
& Ingrid's Invocation Prayer**

FREE DOWNLOAD:

www.WellnessToGo.ca/bookbonus

CREATING

Sacred

Space

A **Journey** to
Self-Healing and
Living the Life
of YOUR
DREAMS!

DEDICATION

I am dedicating this book which has been a labour of love and intense inner learning to two special men in my life. My son Salisu, who came into the world to be one of my many teachers and Carlos Perez, for expressing his love and support by being my cheerleader and patiently rereading and giving insight into every draft I wrote.

Thank you, Thank you, Thank you!

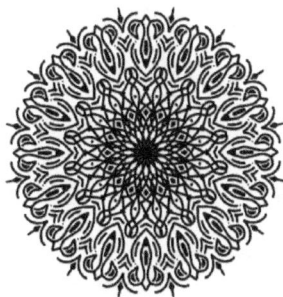

INTRODUCTION

*"The saddest summary of
a life contains three
descriptions: could have,
might have, and
should have."*

—LOUIS E. BOONE

Were you born to live the

life of your dreams?

My answer is YES!

Some may not agree, but I've come to believe that you come into the world already made. This wisdom I gained through observing from the perspective of a mom. I saw my son composed of spirit, energy, and feelings enveloped in likes, dislikes; preferences giving verbal and non-verbal cues before having full knowledge of the world or environment he was born into. For me, my dream was to write a book, but it would take years to discover what type of book I wanted to write! As a young girl, I wrote poetry and art books and pretended I was selling them at famous art and book stores around the world. A very simple dream that I left behind as I journeyed into adulthood and my own process of self-discovery.

It took me two decades to find the commitment to write my book. At first, I procrastinated because I was unwilling to participate in the process of becoming an author; however, over time, my perspective changed, and I realized it could be a fun and enjoyable experience. A friend sent me a poem called *The Assignment* by Layla Saad, which was very appropriate for my process of dragging my feet to take action. It was a nurturing call to slow down and go inwards; an invitation to 'shut out the noise' of distraction and finally focus on fulfilling this non-negotiable need, regardless if I failed or not. Finally, I was going to write the book.

I wrote this book to fulfil a dream and to help those who have some undiscovered awareness; who are in the process of self-discovery; and who desire, want, or resonate with the 'source or infinite,' but are unable to tap into it long enough to find inner guidance.

My hope is that this book will teach you to let yourself 'be' what is already there. There is no 'becoming' since you already are in your entirety. And from that place of awareness that you will choose you, the undeniable knowing in spirit, in feeling, the non-verbal cues that align when things happen. My deepest wish is that this book will bridge the gap step by step and bring alignment of the physical and spiritual journey that pushes you beyond your comfort zone, so you can confidently answer yes to the questions I am asking you.

Were you born to live the life of your dreams?

Were you born to have a great relationship with self, with your innermost awareness of who you are?

Again, I would answer YES!

What stops this process of aligning with your dreams and True Self? Our inability. The definition of inability is the state of being unable to do something. Our inability to take action on our intuition, on our thoughts, on our passions, on our desires, on our commitment to making changes.

The purpose of this book is to help you learn how to act on your intuition and stay in a habitual state of connecting with your True Self. **The best possible version of yourself comes when your spirit and mind complement each other**. Allow me to encourage you to take action and use this book to build and create the best possible version of yourself!

MY JOURNEY

For close to a decade, I lived in a permanent health crisis that cost me jobs, friendships, and relationships. I had what I called a half-life. Eventually, I found my breakthroughs in my healing, which led me to develop my own personal practice of Sacred Space.

Drawing on more than 15 years of experience as an expert holistic health practitioner, reiki master, health coach and speaker I've used these life lessons to help my clients find joy in their relationships, more fulfillment in their careers, and transition through illnesses with partners and family. They've learned to manage overwhelming emotional and physical crisis while continuing to have a healthy positive outlook on life.

*"The best way to predict
your future is to create it."*

—ABRAHAM LINCOLN

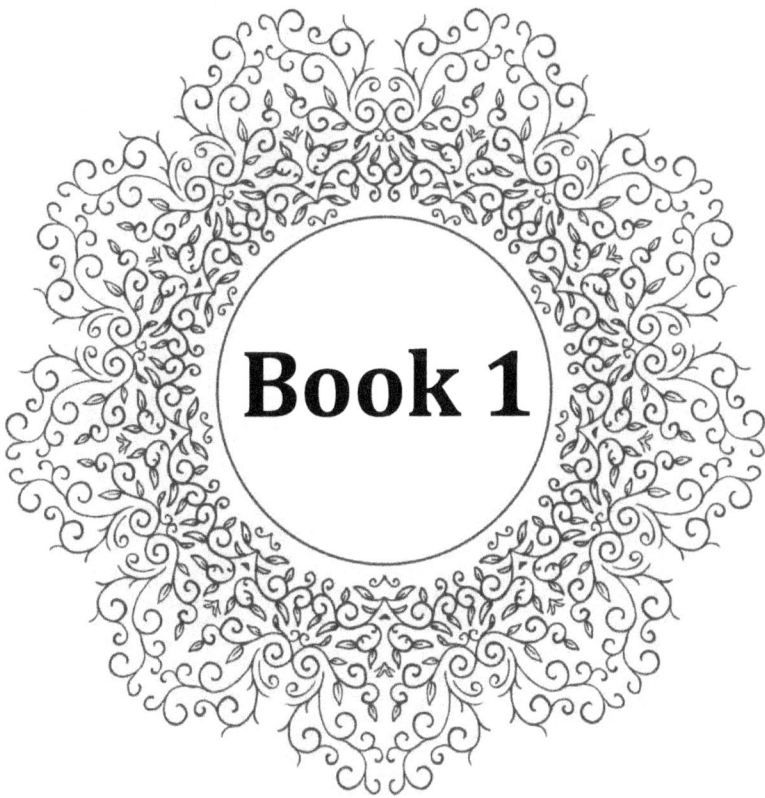

Book 1

ACTING ON YOUR INTUITION

*"Look at the sky.
We are not alone.
The whole universe is
friendly to us and conspires
only to give the best to those
who dream and work."*

—A. P. J. ABDUL KALAM

INTUITION AND SACRED SPACE

Sacred space is the practice and acknowledgement that you are 'source'; your True Self. This is a concept that connects us to our inner knowing of what's inside of us; our soul. Sacred space can be used as a tool to develop your confidence to take action on the feeling or the message you are receiving and tune your intuitive skills to work better for you. Through using this practice, you can build your self-assurance to act on these feelings, messages, and insights with ease.

Intuition is all feeling. There is no rational or conscious reasoning––you are, you do, you step into being with an innate awareness. Your intuition doesn't have conversations with you, you just feel what you know, and you know what you feel, there is no dialogue, there is only instruction that follows the feeling state. Your only task is to act on the feeling or the message.

I had a client years ago who was a successful business professional. During our consultations he shared one of his secrets that he practiced that helped him accomplish some of his success. He said that he made it a habit to repeat a few phrases, one of which was "I believe, I believe, I believe" as he interacted with clients and colleagues. He said this practice helped him to follow his gut instincts on deals, showed him how to avoid problems, and even when it was time for him to go after his dreams and ambitions. The "I believe" helped him to trust his inner knowing even when there was no obvious reason to do so. He shared that he drew on this feeling because "it gave him a sense of peace and courage."

WHAT IS SOURCE?

For me source is the infinite presence within us, also referred to as the unseen soul self or the True Self. The feeling state that we experience every day but we're unable to see physically.

Knowing that you are a source; the source, empowers you to be more than just your physical limitations.

The meaning of this is simple; when those feelings expand into clear thoughts and emotions you can take more aligned deliberate action with source, and in that moment, you are in direct communication with your True Self. This alignment means that what you think and how you act are the same. You are able to go beyond what you are seeing or experiencing physically. For example, a circumstance that may appear impossible to others but feels very hopeful and possible to you. And because of this feeling of hope you take action and or make decisions that align with your True-Self feelings. Just like my client who acted on feelings that helped him to close deals, avoid problems, and be successful. Once you embrace this new belief or knowledge of the existence of source within you, you can connect easily with your other senses, which in turn gives you additional feedback that you can use to help clarify your feelings and actions that you will take in accordance with your True Self.

What you discover here is your keen intuitive awareness that helps you to perceive through sight, touch, hearing, smell, and taste; subtle important messages meant just for you. As you become more comfortable and attuned to this feedback of information, your senses are heightened and begin to culminate into a higher development, to become what is known as your sixth sense. **You now have the merging of source; your True Self and intuition working in tandem together for the benefit of you!**

CREATING SACRED SPACE

There are three aspects of sacred space. The body, the soul, and the mind. All three can be developed individually or together. Your intuition merged with your True Self plays a key role in helping you become and stay aware of the needs and development of each of these aspects. For example, cultivating sacred space for the body may include movement, or a sound practice such as singing or drumming. The soul may include a silent or vocal mantra meditation, and the mind may include autosuggestion or affirmation practices.

Body – Physical sacred space (health, career, relationships)

Soul – Spiritual sacred space (inner journey, enlightenment, evolving)

Mind – Mental/emotional sacred space (disciplining of the mind, emotions, and behaviour)

Through the process of experiencing and creating sacred space, **you will learn the practice of how to merge source; your True Self and intuition working in tandem together for the benefit of you!**

The process requires you to be authentic and vulnerable with who you are; you are face to face with your True Self; your source. You are asked to be plain and transparent, be open, this is the place and time to be honest because only then can you receive the answers to exactly what you need. You will have the opportunity to grow and transform mentally and spiritually as you gain the aptitude to use this feedback from the True Self and intuition. As you take deliberate action with the process you will no longer be motivated by fear or doubt of the unknown, you will learn to practice and work as a team.

You can now replace that old motivation of fear with a new one that is governed by compassion and love through the True Self. This change can bring about that sense of peace and courage, which my client expressed, and it gives you the opportunity to have this with each new experience. With this new awareness, you can now identify how these emotions of compassion and love can guide your behaviors for better outcomes using your intuition and True Self.

The Benefits of Creating Your Sacred Space Practice

You will develop a heightened awareness and gain confidence in your own abilities to assess your physical, mental, and soul state, and in doing so be able to use it effectively to assist you in your everyday life. Sacred space practice can be used before interviews, after a toxic confrontation, an argument or a difficult interaction. You can use it to regroup, get clarity of mind, to ground you in the physical body when feeling not yourself, to get a different perspective on a situation, to help with manifestation practices, to create abundance in your life, to benefit your mental state before meetings, after meetings, planning and managing projects, studying for students and teens, healing emotionally difficult situations, and overcoming trauma.

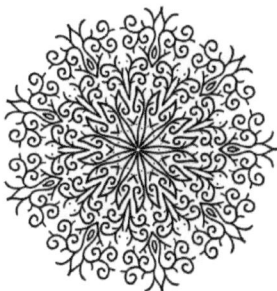

DISCOVERING YOUR SOURCE

"To enjoy good health, to bring true happiness to one's family, to bring peace to all, one must first discipline and control one's own mind. If a man can control his mind, he can find the way to enlightenment, and all wisdom and virtue will naturally come to him."

—BUDDHA

LETS BEGIN

It is necessary to do this once per day or once per week; however, the important thing is consistency, so decide how much time you can give and the best time of day to do it. Eventually it should be done a few times per week until it becomes an easy thing to do as part of your emotional support practice.

Tone and Intention

First set the tone, this is a general overall quality of the moment. It could be simply choosing a dominant thought to say, such as "I feel amazing," or wanting to change a feeling, such as moving from frustrated to having courage, so you would say, "I am connecting with my feelings of having more confidence and courage right now." Next, set the intention, this is the aim or the planned destination based on what you are seeking in the moment. For example, when I'm teaching a yoga class I might say, "Let's set the intention to commit to letting go, or let's commit to facing our inner truths." You might say, "I set the intention to have a great meeting, presentation, or to be more patient and wait for right timing." The purpose of taking the time to do these two steps of preparation is to begin the learning of policing your awareness. What's going on in your mind? What are you feeling and how do you take the steps to change it if you don't like what you're focusing on? The key thing to understand is sacred space is not a religious practice, it is a ritual practice. This means you will follow an order of actions, and these actions are the process necessary to help you develop your deeper awareness of the three aspects of body, soul, and mind.

Setting

Depending on where you are and when you choose to do your practice you can sit or stand to open sacred space.

Now begins the process of connecting with the infinite source that you are and that exists all around you. Acknowledging the four winds also known as the four corners (south, west, north, and east) honors the elements, brings great appreciation and takes the time to commune with your True Self. You simply call to each direction by name saying "calling the winds of the south, west, north, and east."

To raise your vibrational level or connection to the moment, you will need to repeat a few things repeatedly. Choose to say a few things you're thankful for, you can chant a mantra such as "OM" because it is easy to say, or a prayer that resonates with you. I've included one that I've written as a place to start. Take a few minutes to be silent and go within as you connect with stillness. The steps of calling in the winds, saying a mantra/prayer, going into stillness needs to be repeated a few times to start opening your experience and developing your skill set. My client kept saying, "I believe, I believe, I believe" because it connected him to source; his True Self while functioning in the physical state, he felt more connected and supported when he spoke or closed a deal. The more comfortable you become with repeating your sayings or prayers the more connected and supported you will feel within your physical experiences outside of your practice.

To finish you simply say, "*I am closing sacred space.*"

"*It's not what you are that holds you back, it's what you think you are not.*"

—DENIS WAITLEY

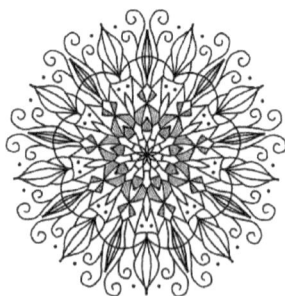

INGRID HERBERT

PRAYER
I am LIGHT

*I am LIGHT, I dispel all
insecurities and fears within
me. I am filled with my
complete beingness in this
moment and I embrace my
full potential to be who I am
perfectly. I am filled with
the unconditional power of
love as I speak my truths
and positive intentions into
today. I shine my light
fearlessly into the world and
stand my ground to utilize
my self-reliance, I trust my
intuition, and I embrace my
inner power. I am not afraid
for my light to shine
brightly throughout the
world today.
And so it is.*

—INGRID HERBERT

There are additional benefits to actively using sacred space to assist you in your everyday life. You can ask for answers to issues, assistance in meetings, presentations, promotions, feel a deeper sense of connection, or ask for direction in a specific area of your life. Being in sacred space is not passive, it is a *doing* state. The more you *do* the more connected you become in the journey, the more is revealed to you, and the more you grow in your True Self. I like the term *get in the game,* you show up to participate.

The practice of sacred space is belief in action. You learn to have synergy with your verbal and non-verbal intuitive messages with complete uniformity. This complementary energy allows for what we do not see, all the aspects of various tasks, the effects of events on others, how to fit lives and situations together in order to benefit the whole, with the efficiency of completing several things at once, meeting all the demands of the emotional, physical, and spiritual needs of all concerned including oneself.

For those of you who would like to go deeper with a spiritual awareness of this practice, here is an example of what I do. I open my space with the tone, intention, and visualization of what I want my outcome to be. Next, I might smudge with an incense such as sage or my own personal mixture, as I continue to focus on the tone and my clear intention. Sometimes I light a candle and chant various mantras, this may be done out loud or in silence. I was once told by a yogi that silence is more powerful, but I find them both equally effective based on the feeling state I want to be in or the feeling state I am already in once I start the process. I do the four directions of the compass, turning to face the actual direction such as east, facing the east. I follow the sequence of the Peruvian Shamans invocation prayers––South, West, North, East. I end with a salutation of prayer, my palms are open, and words of gratitude, always with gratitude.

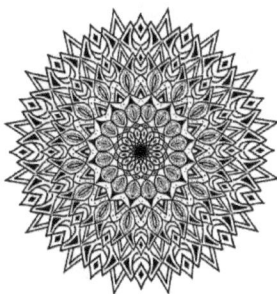

INTUITION, DETOXING AND DE-CLUTTERING ALL AREAS OF YOUR LIFE

"Each morning we are born again, what we do today is what matters most."

—BUDDHA

WHY YOU SHOULD DETOX AND DE-CLUTTER?

D etoxing and de-cluttering brings clarity and focus. There are numerous studies on detoxing for the body that show benefits such as less pain, better functioning organs, and even mental clarity, which I've personally witnessed in my practice with my clients. In this instance, detoxing and de-cluttering is based on your mind and environment. **As you develop the**

practice of sacred space, you need to create order. To do this you need to understand how to let go of the things that are affecting your ability to connect you to your intuition and your True Self.

I usually say to my clients that source is not chaotic. It strives to bring order as it expands and changes on a daily basis, this is also a description of what is known as creative energy. This creative energy can help you with new ideas or being flexible with those daily unexpected changes. You will experience your life expanding and changing as you begin the process of creating order in it. So, it's natural for me to see and I would also want you to see that source is built on what is called an organizing principle. The organizing principle for creating sacred space is built on the understanding of how to create and maintain order and flow in your life to keep it from becoming chaotic. You now know that the practice you're developing includes repetitions, therefore a beginning, a middle, and an end. So, there is a clear direction to guide you if you lose your way within the process of developing this practice around you and within you.

To create order means that you will remove unnecessary things from your mind and environment such as toxic relationships, words, patterns and habits in your behavior that do not complement the best possible version of yourself. Maybe your life feels hectic right now, or you're having difficulty managing family and career, or maybe you've gone back to school to pursue a new career. Whatever the reason in your present environment, the first thing that needs to be done is to detox and de-clutter your mind and environment, so they are working complementary for you.

Detox and de-cluttering are also known as cleansing. Cleansing should happen on a daily basis. We are constantly receiving and sending vibrational messages. Our thoughts, the thoughts of others, our senses, the changes in our emotions affect our every waking moment. Whether we are consciously acting on our thoughts or not, we are making choices and decisions that determine our next action or inaction that we are going to take. So, we take action through the intuitive and True Self as our guide. This guidance helps us to make room for useful things, better experiences, excitement, cheerful energy, in order to reconnect to the energy that is already you. You will get the immediate feedback from the True Self and the sixth sense with the subtle important messages of what needs to leave your life experiences; the things that are not working in tandem for your benefit and self-development, and what should stay in order to cultivate the best version of yourself.

WHAT YOU SHOULD DETOX AND DE-CLUTTER?

We remove toxic relationships such as partners that don't support our vision or friendships that drain our energy, or work colleagues that are disrespectful or condescending to name a few scenarios of where you could start to reflect on. The thoughts that you are thinking on a daily basis are also a good place to start. Do you repeatedly say good things about yourself in your mind? If someone were to tune into your mind and hear what you were thinking right now or your first thoughts in the morning, for example, would you be OK with what they heard?

It is important to detox and de-clutter or cleanse the words and thoughts that are toxic in your mind because they affect how you feel and relate to yourself. Your True Self comes from a place of compassion and love for yourself, therefore you will experience a misalignment with any thoughts and feelings that don't reflect this. You will feel out of sorts or unsure of yourself, you will definitely not have the courage to take action on your intuition for those better outcomes that you are hoping for on your life journey. The key thing that I want you to hear is how this process is about YOU and how YOU RELATE TO YOURSELF. This is very important as you develop a positive, meaningful relationship with your True Self.

> *"I do not fix problems.*
> *I fix thinking.*
> *Then problems*
> *fix themselves."*
>
> —LOUISE HAY

The tool to help you know what you should detox, and de-clutter is effective decision-making. Detoxing and de-cluttering brings clarity and focus. The benefit of this is that **you are present to enjoy an environment that supports you and the way you think and feel.**

As we were growing up, we were told to pick up after ourselves, clean up our messes, and put things back where we found them, in other words, we were being told to put things in order. This is an example of our first introduction into making decisions. Where to put what, do we keep something or throw it out because it's garbage? We had to make very clear decisions regarding the environment in order to bring it back to functioning working order again. And as we know, it would start all over again the next day. You may look around your life right now as an adult and see areas that are in a mess or a slight disarray; areas that do not please you. Let's say your life is like a garden with different sections such as vegetables, rose bushes, a sunflower patch, and herbs. Each section is tended to in different ways because they all have different needs.

As you read this section, you may want to let go of all the things that are not working right now, all at once. But this approach may leave you feeling stuck and indecisive. You may also experience the fear of making the wrong decision. But the truth is your process starts with making one decision at a time. This brings us back to the feeling of the intuition and True Self-acting as one or in tandem. This is your guide your internal compass. The one decision at a time comes from you checking in with what you're feeling intuitively and allowing the deep inner message from the True Self to help you take action on what to do next. It will feel aligned and there will be a sense of peace and courage to support the decision.

This is very different from having contradictions and misalignments in your thoughts that create a cluttered environment. The result of this is you don't take sincere action, your thoughts are scattered and you over promise, and under deliver both to yourself and others. This practice becomes destructive to your relationships and takes you further away from living the life of your dreams. You are disconnected from your True Self and unable to hear your intuition. When you release this resistance of misalignment in your emotional experiences, this helps you to create order and structure in your life again. You become clear with your behavior, your thoughts, and you are able to balance your energy more easily and efficiently. You will feel like yourself again.

The practice of cleansing your mind and physical environment also helps you to develop and create an openness to your energy field to attract the right opportunities and manifestations that you desire. When this happens, you are seen energetically brighter to others, people perceive you differently, and your intuitive instructions are clearer and aligned with your wants and desires.

The following are exercises to help you detox and

de-clutter and cleanse all areas of your life.

Exercise: The Decision Maker

Two tips to making successful decisions every time!

- Be truthful with the outcome you want. This sets your intention and you're able to check in emotionally and move your feeling sense to match your desired outcome

- Ask the question: ***"Am I prepared to do the necessary follow through?"***

Once you're aligned with this way of thinking, you can then go ahead with confidence in making your decision. By the way, you must also be prepared to go ahead with the follow through, which would consist of your True Self and intuitive messages.

Exercise: Cultivating Your Life Garden

Looking at your life like a garden, you might section it as your personal, career, self-development, family, and spiritual journey. Use this as an example to name the section(s) that apply to your needs. Next, identify the area(s) of your garden that are not working or not growing well and write this list on a sheet of paper as your reference. You are now ready to go in and pull out the weeds, water the soil, and nurture the section(s) that are not growing well. This is the process of detoxing and de-cluttering all areas of your life.

PULLING OUT THE WEEDS

Identify conversations you need to have, skills that you need to learn, apologies you need to make, forgiveness that needs to be done, patterns or obligations that are physically killing your joy or disconnecting you from self-healing or inner happiness. List these with the corresponding reference sections of your garden from above and determine the timelines to get them done.

A friend of mine told me that he carried a coin in his pocket to help him with making decisions. He was very indecisive and would get stuck going back and forth with what he should or shouldn't do. One side of the coin said, "Do it", the other side said, "To hell with it."

Now, of course, this is not the most effective way to make an authentic True-Self decision, and for him eventually he had to face the challenges with a bit more thought and practice in becoming a better decision maker. The point is there is no magic to this. There are no short cuts, there is no one pill that will fix it all. You will have to face each decision with transparency and honesty. You will need to nurture and cultivate your life garden to help it grow and thrive in all sections, where all your needs are being met with compassion and love.

Exercise: Tool of Quieting the Mind and Emptying

Quiet your mind so you can start to identify words and thoughts that are toxic to your inner environment. The skill you develop here is how to police your thoughts so that you can stop cultivating the negative and start to nurture and cultivate the positive True Self. This tool assists with de-cluttering so you can hear your intuitive instructions clearly. You get immediate feedback because a quiet mind is similar to a blank canvas. This helps you get to your next emotional decision easier, you are able to develop your connection to your True Self.

Simple 30-Second Breathing Exercise To Help Quiet The Mind

- Connect with the breath going in and out of nostrils only
- Inhale hold for 4 seconds, exhale for 4 seconds

Emptying is also a tool for preparation. Your destination is to create from a place of unlimited possibilities instead of creating from a place of fear, doubt, and negative thinking. Picture a glass filled with water, you take the glass and pour the water out... the act of emptying is the process of pouring the water out. Inhaling and exhaling could also be used to explain the process of emptying, every time you exhale you are pouring the water out, when you inhale the glass fills up again, with your thoughts, emotions, attitudes, situations, etc. It is a process that is constant, like breathing, and like breathing it is essential that you continue to do it to stay alive. Emptying opens you up to welcoming thoughts of inner alignment, contentment, and fulfillment; it introduces you to stillness. In this stillness you will commune with your True Self, you begin to see how the placement of your thoughts affect how you feel. It keeps you open to flow, possibilities, ideas, lightness of being. It is essential because it is continually making space for you to receive and grow, to stay connected to source, to not get stuck with the past, to keep moving. It is not a process of questioning what has happened to you or to delve into your experiences it is simply the act of constantly releasing in order to be prepared to receive. You can only hold your breath for a limited amount of time, eventually you will need to exhale, similarly you will need to pour the water out.

Materials: Sheets of paper or dissolvable paper, pen or pencil

Instructions:

Choose a 5 to 10-minute block of time and write whatever comes to mind, do not reread this, it is not journaling. Once completed shred, tear into pieces or burn paper or place dissolvable paper in water and allow the emptying.

The practice of quieting the mind and emptying prepares you to easily practice letting go.

Exercise: Letting Go

The practice of this is to address specific thoughts or conversations that are stuck in a loop in your mind. You're unable to stop thinking about them or relive doing it differently all the time. For instance, you may have regret about a circumstance, this is the tool to help you let go and move on.

Write down on a sheet of paper thoughts, words, and situations that you consciously need to let go of, again don't read it. Then shred it or tear it into pieces. Do this as often as you need to until you observe yourself no longer thinking about these particular things. A great time to do this is before going to bed.

AFFIRMATION: I let go and create space for the best of what each day has to offer for me.

There is a practice called an action of faith; for example, buying a lamp for your desk at your new job even though you haven't been hired yet, or booking a trip for two with you and your partner even though you're currently single.

These are called actions of faith because you are doing the action based on complete trust of the unknown, but your belief is so strong that there is no room for doubts of the outcome you want. An action of faith that you could do right now to reinforce your de-cluttering would be to physically remove something from your environment that is no longer useful in your life but connects you to an outcome you want in the future; or have a conversation that clearly expresses what you are truly ready to release from a relationship based on how you want the relationship to evolve. When you let go of what you don't want, you will be left with only the things you want in your environment, your mind, your body, and your awareness. This will automatically help you to live only your highest joy as your moments are perceived with more heightened awareness, appreciation and love.

"I learned that maintaining comfort may be easier and safer, but it doesn't often result in what is best for you. If you never feel uncomfortable in your life and career, you are undoubtedly limiting your opportunities to do greater things than you might (ever) have imagined."

—DAVID VAN ROOY

Daily Disciplines That are the Key to Making Positive Changes in Your Life

When we are clear about habits, beliefs, and core values that are healthy for us, this supports the clarity and focus of our environment that is now filled with all the things that we want. I consider this a strong foundation to work from every day because you will feel aligned, safe, and supported as you act on your intuition.

Beliefs, habits, and core values are constantly reinforced consciously and subconsciously over and over again within our thoughts throughout the day, this is the foundation that we work from every day of our lives. In her article *Seven Beliefs of Emotionally Healthy People*, Ellen Hendriksen, Ph.D. writes beliefs such as "I can do things I don't feel like doing, or I can stay the course ...to accomplish goals, and I am capable", are all beliefs that can help you to go a little further such as staying calm in situations that may be pushing your emotions. This means that beliefs can be used as a measure as to where you are and where you want to be with a specific belief or adapted to support the inner alignment with your healthy core values.

The daily discipline is to practice habits, beliefs, and core values that support your internal and external environment. This practice aligns with your True Self and intuitive messages that reinforce the synergy of working together. In your detoxing and de-cluttering, you have taken a close look at the areas, conversations, and ways of thinking that you are now willing to change as you create order in your life. This disciplining is important in learning to have synergy with your verbal and non-verbal intuitive messages with complete uniformity. This complementary energy connects to source that we do not see and also with our habits, beliefs, and core values that could be blocking us from intuitive messages.

As you've cleared your environment let's take a closer look at clearing the mind. Our thoughts are made up of beliefs, these beliefs create habits and they may also connect back to your core values. They all play a role in governing your life. In order to be left with the beliefs, habits, and core values that you do want, first let's identify the beliefs, habits, and core values that are not serving you or that are not helpful in supporting you.

Exercise: Identifying

What are healthy beliefs, habits and core values? The answer will be different for each person.

Examples:

Healthy core values: being accountable, valuing relationships, respecting time, people, and yourself

Healthy beliefs: "I am deserving," "I see the best of what life has to offer," "I have a deep appreciation for myself and others"

Healthy habits: doing the important things first, making your bed, not procrastinating instinctive feelings, expressing emotions and not suppressing them, taking action on your goals

On a sheet of paper write down any thoughts, habits, and self-sabotaging behaviour that is being repeated in your life.

For example, "I overextend myself," "I hide from my dreams," "I am self-conscious and fearful of what others might think if I really did what I wanted to do in my career."

You need to use this to find the clues that will help you replace these thoughts, habits, and behaviours with right thinking. This will serve as a guide to meeting your needs and help to rebuild a healthy sustainable foundation.

First define your core values, then what beliefs support them, and finally create the healthy habits that will reinforce these in your life.

For example, having a core value of a healthy lifestyle would include the belief of choosing healthy foods and experiences that reinforces this through behaviour such as going to the gym and eating at restaurants with healthy menu choices. Once you've identified these three areas, it is time to take action. You are now ready to put the synergy of core values, beliefs, and habits into making those positive changes in your daily life. Once these daily disciplines are in place in your life, you will have beliefs that support your core values to create better inner alignment. You will experience a life with fewer internal contradictions, thus helping you make decisions with deeper awareness and giving you the ability to manage your life with ease. Your healthy habits will be practiced without much effort because the personal reward is so strong that it influences the discipline of your consistent behaviour. The subconscious mind is reinforcing the positive outcome you want at all times.

There is a genuine feeling of accomplishment because your internal and external read on your behaviour is in sync and aligned with your daily experiences. Therefore, it keeps track of your progressive flow of accomplishments. You're either experiencing improvements with maintenance of life being better or you remain neutral with nothing changing in that moment. It is important to understand that your core values are always influencing who you are in the background of your awareness.

Exercise: Trusting Your Intuition; Your Gut

For the next week, you will act from a place of doing. What does your gut tell you? For example, should you speak to the person/stranger on the bus, in the elevator? Should you call that long-lost friend? Whatever you're guided to do act on it (within reason, of course). Journal your experiences to assess how connected you are becoming to your intuition, then make adjustments based on your findings.

TRUSTING YOUR INTUITION

Accelerating your results would start with your awareness of trusting your intuition. Do you trust your gut feeling, and are you able to act on the first message it gives you? Most of us need to have the feeling repeated a few times before we hear or understand it. Unfortunately, this affects timing in our big picture with missed opportunities and setbacks that when looked at in hindsight could have and should have been avoided.

AWARENESS OF YOUR INTUITION

It's a big step, but once you commit to following your intuition your life is more aligned with meeting your needs and keeping you connected to your desired outcome. My personal experience has been that your intuition is right, it knows things you don't know or are unaware of, it's a great guide to lead you in the best direction for that moment.

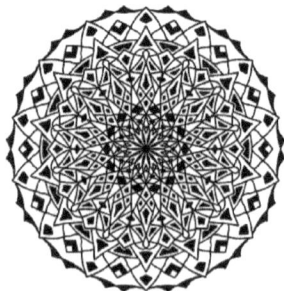

SELF-HEALING

"Even though you may want to move forward in your life, you may have one foot on the brakes. In order to be free, we must learn how to let go. Release the hurt. Release the fear. Refuse to entertain your old pain. The energy it takes to hang onto the past is holding you back from a new life. What is it you would let go of today?"

—MARY MANIN
MORRISSEY

With each stage of self-healing, starting with my body, I would experience huge setbacks that I later learned were directly related to my lack of mental awareness.

Once I discovered how to align my thoughts with my physical healing, I had fewer setbacks and more breakthroughs. I started to get permanent shifts in my healing.

While studying to become a Shiatsu therapist I finally connected spiritually to the practice of meditation, although it took 6 painful months of mandatory 10-minute meditations with my instructor, which I dreaded with every cell in my body. My breakthrough came as a rush of energy into my awareness with one particular meditation where I could see the invisible other side so clearly. I felt rewarded through answers I received in that moment to help with immediate situations I was experiencing at the time.

The answers to your self-healing are within you, you just need to unlock and discover where its hidden itself. The key is found in your awareness. The practice of awareness will open you to rediscovering the process, your unique process of synergy within your True Self.

For me self-healing refers to three key areas, the body, mind, and soul. I believe healing these three areas leads to self-mastery. This is the ability to assert the True Self over oneself in order to be completely and complementary aligned. This asserts a healthy relationship to each aspect of who you are; therefore, the lines of communication between the body, mind, and soul are trusted, non-judgmental, followed, acted upon, and always positioning you in the best possible experience.

THE BODY

My first introduction to self-healing was related to my health issues as a teenager. I found myself at the age of 15 on a quest to find answers to my problems that started at the onset of my first period. I read books on natural healing, I fasted, I experimented with alternative approaches to alleviating debilitating pain and other symptoms that medical doctors were attempting to fix and regulate with medication.

At this stage I was convinced that once I healed my body all other aspects of my life were automatically healed. As I evolved in my body awareness and began to heal, I discovered the disconnect in my mental state of my mind. For example, at times my body felt great and my mind was in a bad mood, this created setbacks because I was unable to sleep and eat, which made me tired, my nervous system became overworked and my pain flared to unbearable heights. These experiences lead me to search for better ways of thinking.

THE MIND

The second stage of self-healing came at the age of 18 when I read the book *The Power of Positive Thinking* by Robert Schuller. Making myself over––this was focused on changing my mental state––the first time I attempted this knowingly was after reading Schuller's book. I had never considered how my thoughts directly affected the health of my body. I began to police my thoughts from that moment on, it took years of practice, but it made a positive difference with my physical healing, the changes stuck, and my body became better as I saw the world with a positive attitude. I later practiced affirmations and autosuggestions to further develop my mental faculties.

THE SOUL

The third and final stage of self-healing came once I began my alternative medicine practice in the 90s while working with clients and their medical and emotional issues. Through developing treatment programs for them, I began to have a better understanding of my personal spiritual development that had started at a very young age with my grandmother's influence, which now played a guiding role of intuition, working with the ancestors and energy medicine that I used in my practice for healing.

What are the areas of your life that need to be healed? Write the answer on a piece of paper. Are you ready to take your foot off the brakes and let go and move forward in your life today? Write the answer of what you would let go of today on a piece of paper.

Exercise: Using the answers from the questions above create a short plan of action that you will start to implement immediately. For example, taking supplements for the body, doing a 15-minute meditation walk each day for the soul, listening to a motivational audio or video twice per week for the mind.

Self-healing requires patience. The patience to wait for your desired outcome with a cheerful attitude, to stay hopeful and with faith.

Here is a tool called *grounding* to help with developing the waiting and staying connected to the desired outcome of healing. Grounding is holding the physical and spiritual space with clarity and intention. Setting an intention of calm and focus becomes the compass that guides you, it also acts as an anchor as you begin to tune into this new shift in the energy of waiting.

As a Reiki Master, I work with my clients' life force energy during their Reiki treatments. This life force energy is simply a vibration, I must ground myself physically and spiritually before I am able to act as a channel to assist with the healing of my client.

To me grounding is a deliberate frequency like tuning into the FM or AM dial on the radio. This vibration becomes a thought, which is then expressed as a feeling, which then materializes into a solution, an action, a word, or a shared experience, eventually it becomes the reality we live in every day. I believe that this process of grounding is a tool that we need to practice and learn, I call it our vibrational tool because it lets us tune ourselves to the right vibration of experiences we want to have. This creates a deeper communion and alignment with your True Self because it lets you live from a place of authentic intention.

Tool for Grounding: Breathe through the nostrils only for 30 seconds to a minute, deep inhales and exhales. Spend 5 to 10 minutes daily writing down your outcomes. Practice patience, have conversations that encourage your waiting in a fun and playful mindset, detach and let go of control of when it should happen, surrender and surrender and surrender to each moment that comes.

Don't lower your expectations to meet your performance. Raise your level of performance to meet your expectations. Expect the best of yourself, and then do what is necessary to make it a reality."

—RALPH MARSTON

OVERCOMING EMOTIONAL SETBACKS

What's a disappointment? What does it look and feel like?

The dictionary says that it is a feeling of sadness or displeasure caused by the nonfulfillment of one's hopes or expectations. Your emotional setbacks such as disappointment, anger, anxiety, fear of success or failure to name a few directly block your ability to hear your intuition and connect you with your True Self, and any one of these emotions could become distractions from accomplishing your end goal in that moment. Mastering your emotional state through your ability to control your mental attitude aligns with your True Self and directly affects the quality of the experiences you will have in your everyday life. Unfortunately, for some of us that moment could last for years, years of being stuck in that emotional state because it plays over and over again in our memory, you are now stuck in the past or the future of this experience. Your conscious awareness of what you will do when you have an emotional setback is your most important step to preventing and overcoming the setback. One of the key things that will help is learning and practicing the habit of disciplining your disappointments.

Exercise: Disciplining Your Disappointments

Learn and practice breathing techniques, count slowly forward or backward and take sips of water to slow your response, the goal is to stay calm, this counters your initial reactions such as anxiety, hurt, and anger with the disappointing experience.

Think forward to your deathbed, what would you say about this disappointment at your funeral in terms of importance in the big picture of your life and your desired outcomes.

Our emotions and sometimes our responses tend to be unexpected and unpredictable, they come out of nowhere, which makes it a challenge to be prepared. However, it is possible to learn certain skill sets that can minimize the effects of the setback in your life. If you're able to keep moving forward and see each moment as de-cluttering the past and entering into a new beginning, this can have a more relaxed effect on the circumstance. We can't control when and how the emotions show up, but we can control how we respond when they do. The feeling-good emotions such as joy, happiness, and gratitude are obvious because it's easy to flow to the next exciting moment when we are experiencing this in our lives. The trick is to connect with this flow of excitement from these feeling-good emotions as quickly as possible when we are experiencing the disappointment from a job loss or not getting a promotion, being frustrated with not accomplishing certain goals in our lives or the anxiety of having a difficult conversation with a loved one or a colleague. The sooner we're able to move past this setback in the moment the sooner we can get to better moments and experiences. We reconnect again to our intuitive messages and True Self guidance of what is the next best action to take.

Asking for and seeking help to move past these setbacks if we're unable to do it for ourselves is very important in building discipline with our mental attitude. Learning how to change our feelings such as anger and frustration to calm and being at ease with the outcome is important to mastering our emotional state and keeping our lives open to better possibilities. This is an area where developing your sacred space practice can help with creating that inner calm, focus, and ease. It will help with learning better ways to respond, such as delaying a response until you have more clarity. Connecting with the flow of excitement no matter what the current circumstance is a valuable skill. It will help you to get unstuck with the uncontrollable factors of the reality you're living in, in the moment. When you develop this ability, you're able to manage your emotions easier, your emotional state and metal attitude are more supportive of the changes or the decisions you need to make.

INGRID HERBERT

SLOW YOUR THINKING

The feet provide easy access to the nervous system because they contain more than 7000 nerve endings. Simply tensing the toes or pushing the soles of the feet into the ground (or shoes) can easily provide a pause and begin the process of calming the nerves. As a reflexologist I've seen how quickly these pressure points relieve tension in the body. Because the entire body is mapped out on the soles of the feet you can stimulate pressure points in the brain to create a body-heart connect for better awareness of what your next steps should be, this leads to creating a calm response internally and then externally through action. This can also be achieved through your hands by putting the palms together and pressing the fingertips.

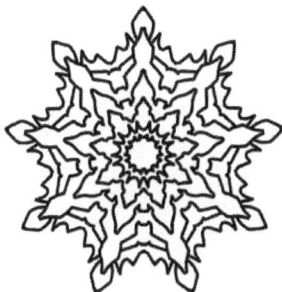

Book 2

HABITUALLY CONNECTING WITH YOUR TRUE SELF

*"Turn on your full potential
– to become no limit, fully
functioning, self-actualizing,
spiritual masters of
your own Destiny. "*

—MARK VICTOR HANSON

HABITS THAT CONNECT YOU TO YOUR PASSION SO YOU CAN START ENJOYING YOUR LIFE FULLY

Wayne Dyer once said, "If you change the way you look at things, the things you look at change." I recently had an amazing conversation with a very special person in my life, and we revisited this concept and where it originates from. The concept is based on the study of matter in its smallest indivisible particle called quarks, which contain fractional electrical charges. Based on experiments that were conducted using an accelerometer, scientists set these particles to collide, and sometimes they found a particle and other times there was nothing. Why this difference, they thought. The answer they concluded was because it is energy, energy that becomes matter or quarks. When scientists analyzed the behavior of the quarks through an atomic microscope, they used light, light is also energy. What they found was that the light affected the behavior of the quarks, they further realized that the quarks' behavior with light and without light were completely different. So, they concluded that when they changed the way they looked at the quarks (with or without light), the way the quarks looked changed. If this is happening on the subtle organic level of matter, then theoretically it should also occur on the obvious larger physical substances such as the energy of the mind and spirit. This behavior of changing becomes intrinsic to energy, meaning it naturally belongs within its state that energy has the ability to change simply by how we see it. If we took this approach to our sacred space practice, we would now have the opportunity to affect our outcomes simply by developing the skills to see things differently.

Your practice of sacred space connects you to your intuitive subtle messages and True Self guidance every day. You would now be able to address and make more deliberate changes to your filters of beliefs, habits, and core values. This would also give you another tool to better manage your daily emotional setbacks by changing how you see your responses or the emotion(s) that triggered them. If you can see this as your new normal, the ability to create change simply by how you see things, you would have a different perspective of how you live your life. This would open your self-awareness to a new belief that it is possible to always consciously be connected to your source; your True Self infinite presence.

This new belief and practice would create a new habit by which this is the only state of being you would act from; you would access your 'joy' or best self with little to no effort. Your alignment with your dreams and ability to act on them would feel like an innate commitment to follow through on your passions and desires and to make the necessary changes with ease. You would begin to answer yes to my initial questions of having a great relationship with self, and with your innermost awareness of who you are.

Exercise: Learning How to Change the Way You See Things

Make a list of a few things that you would like to see differently in your life. Next, write what that difference would look like in as much detail as possible. Because we naturally think in pictures this is a great exercise to develop the pictures we look at on a daily basis in our minds. Therefore, we can easily play with these pictures, and transform them because the nature of energy is to change. When we have fun with energy in a general sense there is no resistance, we just flow, so it is easier to see and make the changes we want to see. For example, you may want a new body image... when you look in the mirror right now, what you see is someone who isn't pretty or handsome, someone who has excess weight, etc. You would then write what you want to see, someone who accepts their body as beautiful, someone who is healthy regardless of weight, body type, or size, etc.

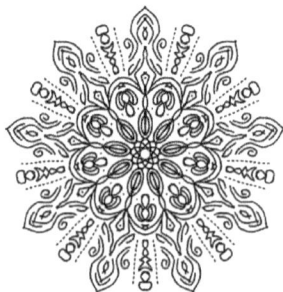

MORE SELF-AWARENESS SO YOU CAN START ENJOYING YOUR LIFE FULLY

There is a Zen Buddhist parable based on the three stages of awakening our hidden potential. The story is that of a young man and his challenges to capture a bull. The young man represents a student seeking, finding and integrating knowledge of the self and the bull represents knowledge. He first searches for the bull or knowledge, on discovering the footprints of the bull he then begins the tracking of the bull; finally he sees the bull or knowledge, at this stage he becomes aware of his own experiences in life. Eventually he catches the bull, which represents his learning of conscious control, his biggest challenge is still to come, which is taming and the riding of the bull. This involves his commitment to practice over and over again his conscious awareness, his perceiving of events and things around him, and eventually integrating the knowledge of the processes he's learning. At this point the story ends with the bull disappearing. The student remains with knowledge transcending to source his True Self. He is now one with his potential and the knowledge that he has the ability of integrating them to work together.

The steps introduced to you in this book are similar to this parable. As you went through the process of creating your sacred space practice, de-cluttering, and learning how to overcome emotional challenges you were seeking, finding, and integrating the knowledge of your True Self.

You were on a path to have a more meaningful life. To connect with your joy, your happiness, you were learning how to make choices based on your decisions and then take the necessary action while staying true to the body, soul, and mind connection integrated with your intuition. You were becoming and developing your self-awareness both internally and externally.

According to this Forbes study, "95% of people think they are self-aware, but in fact the truth is only 10-15% really are" in an article written by Jeff Kauflin. (May 2017)

Mastering your emotional state through your ability to control your mental attitude is a form of self-awareness. If you can choose to see a setback differently by being introspective, ask yourself questions that can give you answers that reflect better choices with your True Self then you can decide what the correct next steps are, and you can better prepare for the impact these decisions will have in your day-to-day life. You can learn deeper self-awareness by practicing over and over again conscious awareness, perceiving events and things around you. The more you practice the more habit forming it becomes. Your deeper self-awareness can only be mastered through that same commitment. You do it consistently by taking a closer look at the impact of your decisions and choices and reflecting on what is working and what is not. Then you make the adjustment to keep the things that are making your life better and let go of the things that aren't.

The emotions of self-doubt and self-judgment tend to keep us out of alignment with our True Self, this directly affects the quality of the experiences we are having in our everyday lives. Because we might second-guess what the right action is to take, even if we are getting strong intuitive messages it can then delay the positive outcomes we were hoping to have. Mastery allows you to experience yourself in present time, your conscious awareness that all parts: body, mind, and soul, are influencing each other and the choices you are making gives you the confidence to not second-guess yourself. You can get ahead of the decision so that the outcome you get is the one you wanted it to be.

Again, like the student in the parable, you must integrate what you are learning in your life experiences that are connecting you to the excitement, purpose, and passion that bring you fulfillment. Your True Self is responsible with its faculties, desires, and purpose, and "allows consciousness to experience itself in physical and non-physical form." (Master Tony) Discouraging inner misalignments such as self-doubt and self-judgement with your thoughts, emotions, actions, and words is a form of self-mastery. It is similar to the student taming the bull. You decide your thoughts, emotions, actions and words that are best to support a life that is more meaningful to you. **When you allow mastery through self-awareness and also consciously practicing the True Self connection, this becomes your habitual state.** You will learn the ability to apply at will whenever necessary the assertion of this state into all your dominant choices, decisions, and actions that you take in your life.

THE HABIT-FORMING PRACTICE

Before you take on a task, any task, make a commitment to be in a high vibration. Why? Because it guarantees a more enjoyable experience. The high vibration I'm referring to is being happy. When we are happy, we manage our disappointments easier, we can push through the setbacks of discouragement, procrastination, or lack of motivation. We are more likely to stay open to our intuition and True Self working in tandem together, giving us the inner guidance we need to make the task easier for ourselves. This ease provides internal and external motivation for us to keep going all the way through to the completion of the task. Another way to look at a task is to see it as your one step at a time. One step at a time could represent health changes you need to make, career choices that need to happen in the next 6 months to a year or the home environment that needs to improve for better communication in your relationship. Taking this approach keeps it small and manageable and you're better able to incorporate your sacred space practice to deal with immediate uncontrollable factors that happen all the time. This high vibration gives you the most optimistic view point for the best outcome and assists you with changing how you see things whenever necessary to keep you moving forward and not become stuck in any setbacks.

You engage your intuitive and your physical

faculties, you are connected to self-confidence, and high self-esteem. In other words, you are committing to winning!

"I believe that everything happens for a reason. People change so that you can learn to let go, things go wrong so that you appreciate them when they're right, you believe lies so you eventually learn to trust no one but yourself, and sometimes good things fall apart so better things can fall together."

—MARILYN MONROE

Exercise: Getting into a High Vibration

Examples: do whatever it takes to get happy using healthy solutions

- Listen to your favorite music, motivational audio/video/podcast (5-10min)

- Breathing in (counts 1,2,3,4) exhaling (counts 1,2,3,4) for 2-5min
- Holding your favorite yoga posture for 30 secs – 1min

Make it a rule of your habit-forming practice to do the thing you don't like doing first, this is based on your priority of frogs that get you to your desired outcome quickly. I discovered this approach when I read the book *Eat the Frog*, by Brian Tracy. Every time you accomplish a desired outcome successfully, you answer yes to living the life of your dreams, you step closer to a more improved future with the possibility to create more happiness in your life. Even though this rule forces you to do the not so enjoyable thing. You instinctively and intellectually know it needs to get done. By taking action you beat your procrastination, it's on your list of priorities to get done so you know you're on the right track, and that feeling of accomplishment will encourage you and give you a deep sense of satisfaction and purpose, which aligns you to do that habit again. It will no longer feel like a forced will power act that you need to push yourself to get through, instead you will experience excitement and desire to be a part of the process of getting it done. This is similar to the stages of the parable with the bull:

you discover and awaken your hidden potential through this regular practice, it starts to become an automatic reaction of self-awareness. You know the way and the reward, so you are more likely to implement another habit that connects you to your passion, and another and so on.

Exercise: Make a list of 'frogs,' the things that if you took action right now would have the greatest impact in your near future in a positive way. For example, making that phone call, planning the day/week ahead, cleaning (desk, closet). You can encourage and develop this even further when you start each day feeling happy. Do whatever it takes to get happy it's an energy that motivates you, you're easily being the best version of yourself, and you have a great personable version of yourself to work with. Have a routine that gets you ready to win the day, a structure that guarantees a great outcome, and prepares you for distractions. This way you're not blindsided by your own self-sabotage and you can easily manage and eliminate setbacks.

Exercise: create a routine(s) that puts you in a position to enjoy your life fully. See the following examples:

- Take mini pauses (breathe, regroup, reset), change your environment.

- Start the morning with a prayer/affirmation/exercise.
- Say to yourself thank you, thank you, thank you, repeat it as a mantra that you say often.
- Be ready at each moment to begin again.

Recap: be in a high vibration, do the thing you don't like doing first, start your day with choosing to feel happy.

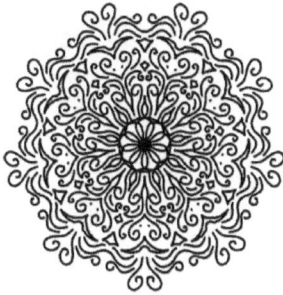

TECHNIQUES TO NAVIGATE THE DAY-TO-DAY AND GET MORE SATISFACTION FROM ACHIEVING YOUR GOALS

TECHNIQUE NUMBER 1:
Check in with your self-awareness

You need to see what is happening around you, how you are interacting with the process to accomplishing your goals. Then go beyond this by observing your internal and external responses, thoughts, and feelings. Use this technique to learn and develop more self-reflection, which will help with aligning you to feel motivated with the goal you want.

Note: You should take small pauses to regroup throughout the day, check in with your awareness to know if you're really doing OK. If something needs to be addressed that you may have missed or forgotten, you ask yourself, "are my actions and thoughts aligned with the outcome of the day?"

Exercise: Set one goal and intention to be achieved for the day or the week. Next, connect with the habit-forming practices to help add the quality of being in a high vibration to your experience so you can begin to build in satisfaction and eventually joy to your achievements.

TECHNIQUE NUMBER 2:
Be ruthless with distractions

Catching the bull took patience and control, it was a process of learning. Similar with navigating your day-to-day so you can live in a more meaningful and fulfilling way and eliminate unnecessary distractions with patience and control. These distractions may come in the form of obligations, guilt, and manipulation by others around you. You must be willing to weed this out of your garden, which you have already started through de-cluttering. This is at your discretion, you would need to identify where and how your time is being wasted or drained by others and then address each situation to align with your needs. Being ruthless with distractions that move you out of alignment mentally, emotionally, spiritually, and physically, helps you to stop the self-sabotage; you don't over promise or under deliver, you are more at peace internally because you are no longer interacting with those situations in your life.

TECHNIQUE NUMBER 3:
Practice Your Core Values

Deciding to practice your core values in everything you do helps you to not struggle with internal contradictions on your thoughts and actions. This contradiction could be you observing yourself saying something to someone but thinking a different thought internally. Having your core values leading the way helps you feel more supported in various situations and events taking place in your life. This transparency keeps you connected to your inner guidance. Because there are no internal contradictions, your thoughts and actions flow creatively with ease to bring new perspectives, viewpoints, and insights.

TAKE IT A STEP FURTHER

When your core values are reflected in your external support systems, such as who you surround yourself with, they align and reinforce your internal focus, which gives you the experience of more satisfaction from achieving your goals. Your expectations are met with ease, no contradictions with responsibilities, no contradictions with reliability. Again, you are in the awakened state with the bull, you have re-established the conscious connection of body and mind with your source your True Self.

ACCELERATE AND ACHIEVE
YOUR BIGGEST GOALS

Exercise: Find and set your own accountability for the life you want to live.

Where are you going to be in the next 5 to 10 years from this moment?

I want you to daydream your answer and once you have clarity write the truth of your vision on a piece of paper or in a journal, be sure that it is what you really want. This vision can be incorporated into your sacred space practice as a part of your future goals.

Note: If you're hesitant or second-guessing while writing this down then you're not in your truth, you need to start again until it flows from the True Self.

Looking at your current situation, list 5 things you would like to keep in your life, list 5 things you would like to let go from your life. Next, answer the question where are you going to be in 5 years if you don't let those things go? What would your current situation look like? Reflect and write your answer. Write this vision of what will happen in your current situation for each of the things that you don't let go. Next, list 5 things that you need to do right now that will get you to where you want to be in your 5-year daydreamed vision.

You are now clear about the steps to take. To accelerate the results you want, you need to check in with your intuition and True Self guidance to be sure that you are aligned with the outcome you want to manifest. To manifest means to show or appear. You are committing to your vision appearing into your life in the next 5 to 10 years.

Moving forward with your steps to accomplishing the big goals will challenge you with how quickly you adjust your emotional setbacks, regroup, begin again and keep your inner alignment stable. These are the goals that sometimes get left behind because they become too overwhelming to manage and you're not able to stay focused all the way to the achievement of them.

You can implement starting with knowing your end goal and what it feels like at the beginning of each day.

When you start with this perspective, you are very clear with each moment as to what is next. You will be able to consistently hold your emotions and pictures in high vibration of what you want. You will experience your thoughts aligning to feed and support everything you want to have happen for the day, even when things go sideways, you won't go with them. Your intuition will guide you with staying consistent with the actions to take to keep your envisioned daydream.

Because your power comes from source and directly connects to your feeling state your aim should continue to be the highest vibration possible. Your visual pictures connected with your vision will aid in keeping your senses activated to also assist with holding this high vibration to help with manifesting your desired outcomes.

You will be guided to know exactly where the work needs to be done, you will develop the connection to change your feelings to match the state you need. Once you are comfortable in this self-awareness, you will be in a mindset of loving compassionate control over your True Self to stay in your power.

Exercise: Autosuggestion Affirmation – Repeat Daily and Often

"I am in my full power. Living from my full potential, exceeding all my expectations, manifesting all of my desired outcomes with ease!"

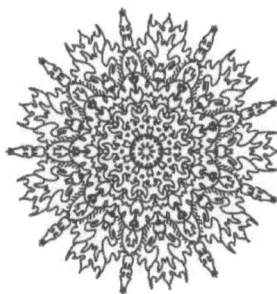

MASTER THE SKILLS TO CREATE THE IDEAL LIFE YOU'VE ALWAYS ENVISIONED FOR YOURSELF

"Before enlightenment, chop wood, carry water. After enlightenment, chop wood, carry water."

—ANCIENT CHINESE PROVERB

A s you can see, the journey has been an internal one. What you think, how you feel, what decisions you need to make, what is your view point, what is your outlook, what do you want for yourself? All of these questions have led to your self-discovery.

Knowing these answers about yourself helps you to be more confidently connected to who you truly are.

As you move forward, you need to remember to not act from the clues of your external reality, which means even if your day is not going as planned don't allow things not working out to disconnect you from your True Self, but to act only from your True Self and instincts to keep your inner alignment focused on the outcome you want to have happen.

> *"Our ambition should be to rule ourselves, the true kingdom for each one of us; and true progress is to know more, and be more, and to do more."*
>
> —OSCAR WILDE

Be flexible in your perspective so you can draw on your strengths in the immediate circumstance and not feel stuck with any limiting viewpoints. These limitations may look like challenges or crisis of not feeling calm and self-assured with what actions to take. You may feel in the moment that it is impossible to connect to your joy or happiness to stay in your high vibration, but this is all the more reason to over prepare for these day-to-day stressors so you can feel comfortable while waiting for the feelings of alignment to become part of your experience again.

MASTERING YOUR ABILITY TO MAKE AN EMOTIONAL CHOICE

Developing your ability to make a deliberate emotional choice, even if you're in the midst of experiencing what you don't want, helps you to keep moving forward out of the circumstance.

Deliberately choosing to feel happy when you are frustrated or choosing optimism when you feel discouraged is the practice of making a conscious emotional choice. It may initially seem like just words because you may not have the feeling, but you are creating your ability to think the way you want to feel. This also helps you to gain access to being guided out of your crisis with the assistance of source; your True Self. This comfortable feeling of being guided out of your crisis helps you to be spontaneous as you remain conscious of your response. Therefore, this spontaneity is part of your connection to your self-awareness and helps you to stay curious, interested, engaged, and free of any debilitating trauma that may come from the challenges in that moment.

ENTERING INTO THE SPIRIT OF IT

There is a statement that comes from the first chapter of *Dore* by Thomas Troward, called "Entering Into The Spirit of It," which explains our ability to constantly keep manifesting from source, newer and better experiences and outcomes if we deliberately choose to do so.

The statement reads: "My mind is a center of Divine operation. The divine operation is always for expansion and fuller expression, and this means the production of something beyond what has gone before, something entirely new, not included in the past experience, though proceeding out of it by an orderly sequence of growth. Therefore, since the Divine cannot change its inherent nature, it must operate in the same manner with me; consequently, in my own special world, of which I am the center, it will move forward to produce new conditions, always in advance of any that have gone before."

You may need to read the statement a few times to truly grasp the concept of how it turns on your full potential and gives you access to mastering your own destiny through source, which is referred to as the Divine. It says '...in my own special world, of which I am the center, it [the Divine] will move forward to produce new conditions...' these new conditions are whatever you see them to be. What new circumstances do you want to live? What challenges do you want to overcome? This is where seeing your pictures differently will directly affect the new circumstances the Divine produces for you to live in.

In this place of mastery, you can become a no-limit, fully functioning, self-actualizing, spiritual master of your present now, where you step into enlightenment and rule over yourself. Mastering chopping wood and carrying water is being in the present now with a de-cluttered mind, self-aware of your thoughts, hearing your subtle intuitive messages, and being guided with decisive instructions from your True Self. From this place of clarity, all of your actions can be directly linked to your envisioned life, making it the motivation to assess your current reality of any situation so you can make the necessary decisions to change it. Your envisioned life, the ideal life you want to create for yourself needs to be a clear picture that you see every day until every detail becomes the reality you wake up to. Once this happens you are ready to master your present now.

So let's begin...

"I don't allow my faith to become filled with fear."

—ANONYMOUS

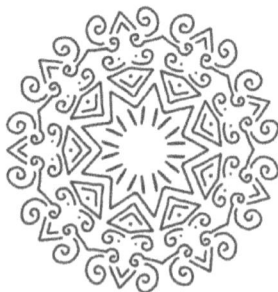

SPECIAL BONUS

As a special thanks for purchasing this book, I am offering you the following bonuses:

Free download of my tools to complement your healing journey:

Detox & De-Clutter 101
and
**The Sacred Space Process
& Ingrid's Invocation Prayer**

FREE DOWNLOAD:

www.WellnessToGo.ca/bookbonus

www.ingramcontent.com/pod-product-compliance
Lightning Source LLC
Chambersburg PA
CBHW030254030426
42336CB00009B/377